COGNITIVE BEHAVIORAL THERAPY

A CBT Guide To Theories & Professional Practice

© 2019 BILL ANDREWS, ALL RIGHTS RESERVED

DISCLAIMER

The author has made every attempt to be as accurate and complete as possible in the creation of this publication, however he does not warrant or represent at any time that the contents within are accurate due to the rapidly changing nature of the Internet. The author assumes no responsibility for errors, omissions, or contrary interpretation of the subject matter herein. Any perceived slights of specific persons, people, organizations or other published materials are unintentional and references are used solely for educational purposes.

This information is not intended for use as a source of medical advice. All readers are advised to seek services of competent professionals in the psychology field.

The practice of psychology requires specific knowledge, experience, and understanding of how to apply these practices. You MUST consult a trained and skilled practitioner in the mental health fields before attempting any of the listed techniques in this eBook.

Further, a psychiatrist should be involved in any or all situations where a formal diagnosis needs to be made as he or she is also a medical doctor and can make decisions based on body physiology as well as mental health.

The information herein is meant to be for the basic understanding of core principles and wherever possible will include footnotes and markers from accredited universities that support such concepts.

.

CONTENTS

Chapter 1: Cognitive Behavioral Therapy In Practice & Uses 1
   The DSM (V) — CBT Exploration Of Potential Uses 3
   The Final Product: Cognitive Behavioral Therapy At A Glance 5

Chapter 2: Cognitive Behavioral Therapy (CBT) What Is It Really 8
   What Is Cognitive Therapy 12
   The Behavior With The Cognition 13
   The Psychosocial Approach Used In CBT 15

Chapter 3: Changing Maladaptive Thinking 18
   The Main Goal Of Cognitive Behavioral Therapy 18
   Cognitive-Behavioral *Assessment Model 20
   Effective Considerations For The Assessment 21
   Intervention & Treatment Analysis 24
   The Power Of CBT: Removal Of Erroneous Thinking 26

Chapter 4: Cognitive Distortions Made Whole 27
   Over Generalizing, Magnifying Negatives, Minimizing Positives and Catastrophizing 31
   Reducing Emotional Distress with CBT 34
   Challenging Maladaptive Thoughts & Destroying Them 36

Chapter 5: Modern CBT & The Latest Tools 38
   Systematic Desensitization 39
   Exposure Therapy 39
   Stress Inoculation 41
   Cognitive Processing 42
   Acceptance Therapy 44
   Mindfulness Based Cognitive Therapy 45
   Meditative Practices 47
   Behavioral Modification (R+) 47

Chapter 6: The 6 Phases of CBT Explained For Therapy Use 50
   Assessment or Psychological Assessment 50
   Re-Conceptualization 52
   Skills Acquisition 54
   Skills Consolidation And Application Training 54
   Generalization and Maintenance 56
   Post-Treatment Assessment Follow-Up 57

Chapter 7: Best Uses for CBT & Beyond 59

Conclusion 62

CHAPTER 1
INTRODUCTION – COGNITIVE BEHAVIORAL THERAPY IN PRACTICE & USE

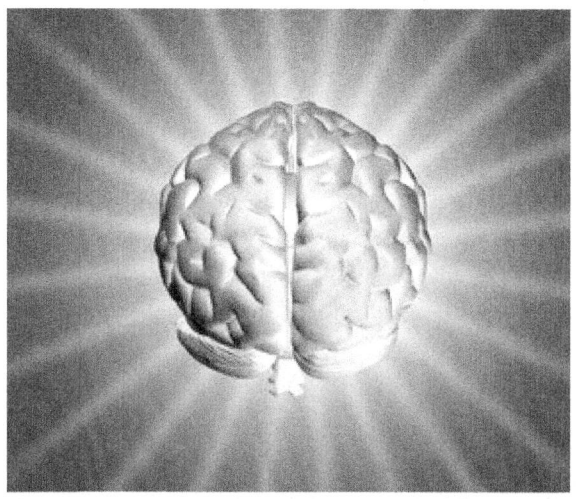

Cognitive-Behavioral Therapy (CBT) is best known for combining knowledge about **how people learn** with **theories about thinking**.

CBT is now considered to be one of the leading, if not the best-established, treatments for many mental health conditions and its practice and use is on the rise.

Dozens of current and past research projects have established its effectiveness, and the skills people learn in CBT continue to help long after therapy is discontinued.

In this guide, we will introduce CBT and express many positive uses for it as a therapy. **While it is important to have a qualified therapist use the verticals in treatment**, many of the cognitive and behavioral tools used to implement it can be learned by the average person to effect change in their daily lives.

There can be little question CBT is now a powerful force for change in people's lives and far superior to many other singular therapies, as it focuses on real world tools and steps to make life better for the individual.

In CBT the relationship between therapist and client is more like a partnership. Client and therapist work together to identify patterns of maladaptive behavior and thought.

Once identified, the goal is to eliminate over time, thoughts and behavior patterns that contribute to dysfunction.

The client and therapist also look at how thoughts can impact behaviors and how the two are related. The causal chain of events is also studied. For example, if a person believes they will fail at almost everything, that belief alone can lead to depression and a self-fulfilling prophesy of isolation, withdrawl from society and increases in failure.

Identifying negative thoughts and the negative reinforcement of these patterns is a primary concern.

In CBT, carefully targeted exercises and even homework are used to help clients see these patterns. The client is then free to implement changes. Contingent on the client's needs, the therapy can then shift to focus more on behaviors or thoughts.

For example, if someone is experiencing avoidance behavior in social situations, the behavior is more targeted than cognition is. If the inverse is true, the client might need to focus on *feelings first* and ways to adjust unreal thinking patterns to reduce negative feelings about themselves.

An additional component of CBT is to identify maladaptive feelings and unrealistic and or negative thinking.

The practice and uses of CBT are wide-reaching and powerful. Properly used, the therapy can confront and control most forms of disorders including many of the top mental health issues in society today.

The Diagnostic Statistical Manual or DSM (5), the current diagnostic manual used by experts in mental health, allows for congruency and collaboration as well as a general consensus that enables health care professionals to agree on basic criteria for generalized diagnostics.

Our first section explores the uses of the DSM in the age of CBT. The two can be used concurrently or sequentially and do not necessarily have to be diametrically opposed to each other.

In fact, if the DSM can add anything to our discussion, it will most likely be a way to reach out to those suffering from core disorders that are agreed upon, and then to apply CBT more effectively. Our final step will be to identify and then treat in steps, generalized disorders as well as active contributions from new emerging therapies where applicable.

Let us explore this possibility.

THE DSM (V) – CBT EXPLORATION OF POTENTIAL USES

One of the biggest concerns with psychopathology is to try to quantify what exactly a "disorder" is. Some people can operate just fine with a suggested disorder, while other potential patients have moderate or extreme difficulty functioning in society.

Thus, the real reasoning for classifying mental disorders is more for practitioners and those who interact with people affected as a way to mainline ideas for therapy.

This also allows us, as professionals, to see the following benefits:

- ✓ ***A common vernacular*** for both identifying and classifying patients even where understanding is not 100%.
- ✓ ***A way to advance psychopathology*** in a language that can be shared with peers and other professionals.

- ✓ ***The advancement of new treatments*** and a way to also classify potential newly identified mental health disorders and communication of related data.
- ✓ ***A generalized tool for treatment***.

Some critics of the DSM have stated that just because PhDs decide to gather and interpret data to create a disorder, does not necessarily mean that it is actually a dysfunction or they suggest that such a dysfunction can be very subjective based on created criteria that are more subjective and contingent on patients and their observable behavior. For example, the DSM defines **ADHD** (Attention Deficit, Hyperactivity Disorder) as:

"A persistent pattern of inattention and/or hyperactivity-impulsivity that interferes with functioning or development."

To further classify a disorder, the DSM also explains that the patient must project a certain number of **symptoms** over a certain time period (i.e. 6 months):

"Individuals with ADHD may present with both inattention and hyperactivity/impulsivity, or one symptom pattern may predominate."

With **CBT** we are trying to first identify disorders. Once identification is accomplished using the DSM, we can see the relational therapies as suggested by other practitioners.

The key is to ***explore not only older therapies but the latest white papers*** and look for the most effective and least intrusive therapy or therapies that both work in conjunction with the disorder.

For example, **ADHD** is often countered or lessened with medication. So, is ADHD really a mental health disorder or more of a metabolic imbalance?

Often the family is impacted by any therapy, and there are

arguments against drugs that seem logical. Yet CBT seeks to focus on **the patient regaining control** typically without drug intervention. The use of drugs is secondary and only considered if traditional therapy fails.

We can clearly see the need for the DSM as a diagnostic tool, but we need **not** be totally constrained by it. Few who practice psychology would argue against the power of the DSM as a tool, yet we need to consider first and foremost the thoughts, feelings, and behavior of the patient during the diagnosis too.

When we do - we offer the very best kind of therapy; one that reaches the patient on an emotional, logical and behavioral level and seeks to help, not always label.

Behaviorist Dr. Skinner would also be the first to remind us that the **ultimate expression of any organism is its behavior**. We need to quantify and then exact control over stimuli for the use of positive reinforcement (R+) for the continuation of any successive therapy. CBT therefore, is not just another therapy but is built on all three factors: feelings, thoughts and finally behavior and ways to modify all three.

When we bring together current, past and present therapies, the correct diagnostic tools and behavior modification, we have almost guaranteed success for helping a patient with recovery and the ability to navigate society successfully.

THE FINAL PRODUCT; COGNITIVE BEHAVIORAL THERAPY AT A GLANCE

Now we can finally see exactly what the intentions of CBT are: a perfect world where the triad of *thoughts, feelings, and behavior* come together to create health and wellness in the individual, and freedom from dysfunction.

Much like the concept of the **yin and the yang**, personal characteristics must be balanced in order to maintain optimal health. Imbalances create disruptions in behaviors and can lead to sickness and disorders.

This is in part the final product of cognitive behavioral therapy; where the patient recognizes the imbalances and works together as a partner with the therapist to correct these imbalances.

Therefore, it is necessary to view **the patient** as containing a form of "snapshot" of their current mental health showing exactly where they are based on diagnostic criteria. The DSM is the main diagnostic tool, but there are also additional tests that can be administered by the psychologist to determine additional dysfunction or problematic areas.

The tests can then be used to further pinpoint possible dysfunction in other areas. The purpose is to bring forth a balance among thoughts, behaviors and those things that precede emotional imbalances. When the three come together it creates a 'perfect storm' of sorts and a more complete picture than just a single diagnosis could.

The purpose of CBT is to bring the very best of all three schools of therapy together. Not only is the final process a well-thought-out and controlled therapy, but the utilization of different schools of thought together and in combination allow CBT to become one of the best overall forms of therapy for whatever the disturbances are.

Of course, this is in **a perfect world** where one can reach deep inside of the patient and extract the information necessary to make proper diagnoses.

This is at best a difficult job unless the patient is fully on board and wishes to work as a partner with the therapist.

Cognitive behavioral therapy is also capable of working with some physical maladies that are an expression of mental illness. It is possible to work **backward** with physical manifestations and make partial corrections while also working with the cognitive aspects of any disorder.

This is what makes CBT therapy unique because the combination of several schools of thought can be used to confront multiple issues. Most forms of mental illness or disruptive behavior can manifest and cause overlapping issues that often need to be confronted simultaneously.

CBT addresses all of these issues and works with the patient in a way that is different from singular forms of psychology.

.

CHAPTER 2:
COGNITIVE BEHAVIORAL THERAPY (CBT) WHAT IS IT REALLY?

We are now at the heart of exactly what CBT should be and seeks to become in a patient's life. The good news is that CBT interventions typically focus on **setting realistic and achievable goals** in a progressive stage of learning that takes place with the patient.

While some therapies do not stress necessarily educating the patient first, CBT seeks to pull the curtain back and remove the mysticism that the psychologist is engaged with so as to make the patient an equal partner in corrective actions and applied therapies.

Typically, there will also be **homework** that is assigned, such as engaging in social activities, assertiveness drills and the like to confront different types of dysfunction.

CBT also stresses different types of tools such as: relaxation techniques, systematic desensitization, behavior modification models and other types of somewhat aggressive but collaborative steps like therapies.

The therapist will also work through active role-playing for situations and suggest how to deal with the **escalation of stress,** for example, social anxiety, which is often at the root of most typical disorders.

CBT also seeks to **identify situations that typically are avoided** but can gradually be approached, as mentioned before with systematic desensitization.

CBT also seeks to both identify and then have the patient engage in **enjoyable activities,** which can include hobbies that can be paired with other essential activities such as exercise, relaxation techniques etc.

CBT seeks to challenge all forms of **negative thinking** by using techniques similar to thought stoppage, and replace negative ideologies with more positive ones.

Feelings are also carefully tracked and linked to certain behaviors so that one can determine negative triggers. This step is avoided typically in some therapies, yet it is absolutely critical for CBT to be effective.

Altering of negative behaviors and substitution with positive ones can also be a gradual function of the therapy. Because the therapist does not need to hide or obfuscate anything from the patient, it is much easier to earn the patient's trust and cooperation.

Because of this, CBT is most effective with almost all types of mood disorders including depression. CBT also has a wonderful track record with people that suffer from addictive and or anxiety disorders.

Using CBT can directly treat personality disorders including eating disorders, sexual problems, and even outright psychosis. This approach can include individual counseling or even group and couples therapy, as again patients are approached on a realistic and truthful level and the therapist is not required to keep information that would be used later, as in some types of confrontational therapy.

The applications of CBT are practically limitless, especially when dealing with **mood disorders** such as depression. Since the therapy is non- confrontational, typically education is the first step, followed by a more active role where the patient decides some of the most important focuses of the therapy.

This sense of empowerment is extremely important because **the client fully understands their symptoms** and realizes that the illness can be controlled and eventually overcome by simply performing certain functions, homework, and activities.

This makes complete sense to the typical person that does not understand the correlations of cognition and behavior necessarily.

For the typical person, the ability to simply focus on tasks necessary to complete recovery makes CBT extremely powerful and useful for the typical layman.

Again, this explains why there are such high-performance rates and success rates with CBT as a therapy.

Treatment strategies often include allowing patients to establish not only structure around daily activities, but to become more aware of the benefits of their structure and to see the positive outcome for activities that they engage in.

Because both the therapist and the patient work closely together to challenge negative attitudes, negative thinking and adverse behavior, there is more of a team feeling where the patient perceives him/herself as almost equal to the therapist; thus, empowering them to further perform the necessary steps to heal themselves.

In areas of substance abuse, CBT can be used to prevent relapses in treating problems, especially with alcoholism. While typically some patients are resistant, for those that are motivated to once and for all remove substance abuse from their life, cognitive behavioral strategies involve behavior modification that can eliminate negative reinforcement.

Learning to identify and then challenge problem behaviors is done in a systematic and methodical way that is much like the OCD behavior in the first place. While not attempting to make any patient more OCD, it is far better that they focus on patterns to remove substance abuse from their life than to allow substance abuse to become the focus.

The exploration of both positive and negative drug cravings is taught in behavior modification and applied to the removal of negative cravings and eventual extinction as a behavior modification tool. This includes a self-reinforcing need for the positive feelings associated with any type of drug abuse, allowing for substitution of alternative natural highs such as exercise and or achievement in life. This makes extinction possible in this light.

CBT even adds an additional vertical which involves self-monitoring to recognize early cravings for alcohol and/or drugs and to use extinction to eventually remove these cravings as well. Behavior modification is powerful here.

The development of **avoidance behavior** is then redirected upon *all negative aspects of addiction* where positive reinforcement then is used to reinforce the necessary good behavior on a graduated scale.

Reinforcement is then focused *intermittently* to maintain progress and can be shifted to full positive reinforcement if necessary.

In the case of substance abuse, both the therapist and the patient work together to anticipate problems and create structures to protect the individual from additional relapse.

Each aspect of CBT therefore, needs to be explored and its benefits, as well as possible limitations should also be discussed.

No therapy is perfect, but the combination or triad of CBT would seem to cover all aspects necessary for a patient to recover from almost all types of dysfunction or mental illness, especially those related to addictive behaviors.

WHAT IS COGNITIVE THERAPY?

> **cog·ni·tive ther·a·py**
> *noun*
> a type of psychotherapy in which negative patterns of thought about the self and the world are challenged in order to alter unwanted behavior patterns or treat mood disorders such as depression.

Most forms of therapy focus exclusively on thought patterns. **Cognitive therapy** as explained above is just one part of CBT.

The founder of cognitive therapy was Aaron T. Beck or Aaron Temkin Beck (July 18, 1921) an American psychiatrist, who is regarded as its father. His pioneering theories are widely used in the treatment of clinical depression.

CBT seeks to expand Dr. Beck's theories and apply them more effectively. While clinical depression is certainly worth treating, the application of cognitive therapy, when combined with behaviors and feelings, works well for the resolution of other forms of disorders and mental illness.

The core concepts of cognitive therapy are: **testing the assumptions of the patient** in a way that is reflexive in their life, and the ability to try and shift the assumptions that lead to different emotional turmoil and negative thought.

The concept is to **target thoughts** that are disruptive to the patient, and explore what thoughts are actually leading to what maladaptive behaviors.

Changing the way the patient thinks should elicit gradual changes in behavior, especially on a subconscious level.

The therapy seeks to work on a behavior that is in conflict with the person's choices in their life. While this is not necessarily the best outcome primarily, you can quickly restore someone's higher levels of functioning while they continue to explore the necessary changes to make their lives positive and eventually enjoyable.

Dr. Beck would focus primarily on depression and would attack what he called *cognitive distortions*. These were errors that were either learned or programmed into a person's thinking that would maintain the depression; especially if it involved arbitrary inferences, selective abstractions or other over-generalizations that would lead to disruptive thinking and the minimization of positive events in the patient's life.

Therefore, **cognitive therapy** certainly has its place when it comes to the application of CBT. Cognitive therapy has the power to alter thinking and therefore alter behavior. Yet when you combine behavior with cognition, the two can reinforce each other and strengthen the patient -- allowing for a more positive outcome.

We certainly appreciate Dr. Beck's contribution, but we also seek to add *the behavioral aspect* so that the two may balance each other. Let us now explore behavior with cognition and why the combination is so powerful.

THE BEHAVIOR WITH THE COGNITION

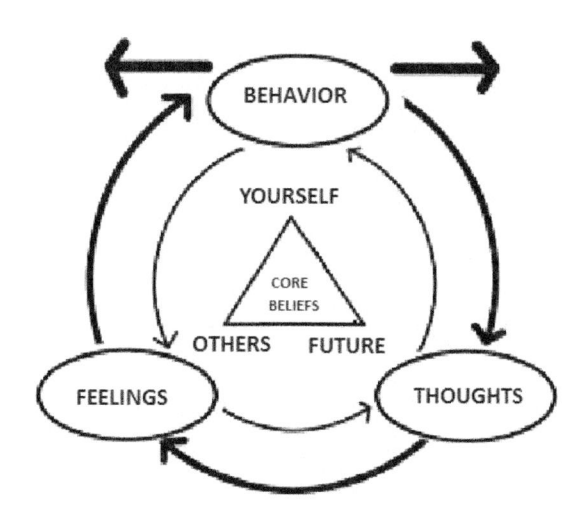

We have skirted around **Behavior Modification** when discussing CBT, but here we will engage it fully and explore how it can be used in conjunction with **cognitive therapy**.

Behavior modification is a unique discipline and is more than just a therapy, but a way to teach both people and even animals (i.e. dogs) how to learn.

Pioneered by **Dr. B. F. Skinner**, the discipline is so much more than a way to control and discipline. Behavior modification proposes that all behavior occurs because it is reinforced to happen. **A primary reinforcer** elicits a response and guarantees it will occur again and again.

For example, a bear in the zoo learns that when the animal steps on a metal pedal near a food chute, it opens and a small treat drops before his feet. **The act equals a reward.** The reward that reinforces the behavior (often referred to as **R+**) is said to be a primary reinforcer if the treat is something that would motivate the animal to repeat the behavior again.

We then get into terms like *intermittent reinforcement* to explain how a primary reinforcer can be delivered occasionally to keep the behavior occurring.

Behavior modification does work well with humans if the primary reinforcer is something they need or want. The core teaching is to create essentially reward-based behaviors that can be used to change negative behaviors.

Differing rewards can be used and this can be anything that the subject values. **Positive reinforcement** (R+) therefore can be whatever a person or animal likes and over time can change to periodic or intermittent reinforcement to keep the new behavior dominant.

With humans, positive attention, the purchase of a new toy or gift, money, pampering or just about any kind of thing can be seen as a form of positive reinforcement that can elicit a positive response.

For example, Joe wants to quit smoking. For each day that he smokes one less cigarette, he puts ten dollars into a shopping fund. When he finally quits he receives the money and can go buy a new guitar, something he really wants.

Behavior modification is then anything that modifies behavior. We create methods to first observe behavior (called a baseline) and then look for stimuli that make the behavior change to the desired outcome.

For example, Steve wants to lose 20 pounds and get in shape, but he can't stop eating Oreo cookies. The cookie is a treat and has become a pleasurable experience and is, therefore, **reinforcing the eating,** which is causing weight gain. Steve needs to find a substitution for the Oreo's pleasurable experience (which is being expressed as a positive pleasurable thing) in order to stop weight gain.

The same can be said for our thoughts. We can reinforce negative imagery that can cause negative instances of behavior to occur.

CBT is in part, a form of Behavior Modification. The term **Cognitive Behavior Modification** (CBM) is the tool as it relates to a systematic reduction of modification of behavior.

CBM (not CBT) is the aspect we are most interested in because this is the expression of the best type of behavior modification as it pertains to CBT. CBT is, therefore, a therapeutic technique that leads to an alteration in negative behavior(s).

THE PSYCHOSOCIAL APPROACH USED IN CBT

The **psychosocial approach** views individuals in the context of how their daily lives are impacted by both others and social factors that can contribute to the overall picture of mental health.

Some of this is based on demands made on the individual and what current coping mechanisms they have.

For example, someone who leads a cloistered or sheltered life does not have the same social demands upon their time as a person living and working in a busy city setting with a job that demands interaction with lots of people.

In one setting, a person requires few coping mechanisms or understanding of ritualized and intricate social inter-workings. In another setting, the demands made on social interactions can be extreme.

It is easy to see how it is sometimes necessary to have a set of detailed skills and coping mechanisms when it comes to dealing with social interaction.

The psychosocial approach in CBT assumes that either improper coping mechanisms or improperly executed social skills or combination of both could be problematic.

Therefore, it becomes necessary for the individual:

- **To learn the necessary coping mechanisms** and/or skills necessary for their unique situation.
- **To leave the individual with the ability to learn** additional coping mechanisms as the need arises.
- **To have the ability to practice coping mechanisms** and/or social interaction in a safe and sheltered environment first.

The essence of CBT demands that the psychosocial approach include the education and learning of various social skills and/or social coping mechanisms.

For example, Lisa often becomes anxious in public and is trying to learn methods for proper stress reduction through breathing techniques that reduce stress.

Lisa first practices these mechanisms until such time as she feels comfortable to execute them in public.

This is a wonderful coping mechanism for Lisa as she has learned part of the cognitive behavioral therapy elicits the ability to control stress and therefore reduces the chances of panic attacks and/or out-of-control anxiety.

We mention this because in future sections we will explain the necessity for learned coping mechanisms and additional social tools necessary for engaging in proper social etiquette.

With learned proper tools and social etiquette, the reduction in mental health issues will continue until the individual is capable of coping with their own environment.

The psychosocial model stresses this process and we wholeheartedly agree that in CBT this is a form of therapy and a necessity for all future interactions.

CHAPTER 3:
CHANGING MALADAPTIVE THINKING

Changing maladaptive thinking is an extension of psychology and one of its core principles. In this section we are going to discuss mainstream cognitive therapy.

Essentially this therapy holds that changes in maladaptive thinking will lead to changes in behavior. While this is true on the surface, there are other important factors to consider that are part of the reason why CBT is much more effective in and of itself than simple cognitive therapy is.

Cognitive therapy attacks cognitive distortions that are causing maladaptive behavior in a person's daily life. For example, the belief that everything a person does will fail is a cognitive distortion and needs to be challenged by the therapist.

Cognitive distortions and challenging the thinking however, are only the beginning of the process. The reason why CBT is so effective is because the main goal of CBT as we will see is all-inclusive and requires interaction and change by the patient.

THE MAIN GOAL OF COGNITIVE BEHAVIORAL THERAPY

Cognitive distortions lead us into the importance of a complete therapy that takes into consideration the final goal of adaptive behavior, as well as the thoughts and feelings of the patient who seeks to normalize their behavior and interact successfully with society again.

As mentioned before, the diagnosis is just the beginning of this process because when most people seek out CBT they are already suffering from one or several disorders that require looking at the person as a whole.

This is what separates basic cognitive therapy from CBT; the ability to deal with the entire person and not just their thoughts. While no therapy is going to exclude the importance of behavior, CBT balances the importance of dealing with cognitive distortions along with behavior and allowing the two to work together in a way that also complements and supports positive feelings and emotions.

This makes CBT not only an effective therapy but one that can continue to grow with the person as they begin to appreciate better thoughts, better moods, better feelings and of course, better behavior.

Where behavior modification falls short, dealing effectively with moods and feelings on a cognitive level can then interact successfully with improved behavior.

This allows the therapist to not only function to address maladaptive behavior but to identify the causal links between cognitive distortions, acting out and the appearance of negative and/or maladaptive behavior.

Therapists are also free to teach patients the importance of dealing with all aspects of their humanity. Extending mental health therapy to people is a process that not only involves cognition but the ability to recognize what cognitive distortions are causing what pain in their lives.

For a person that has grown accustomed to cognitive distortions, it can take some time and even hard work to eventually get to the point to where their behavior begins to change effectively.

This has a very positive impact especially over time when dealing with people that are suffering from various degrees of mental illness.

Some of the more difficult and painful behaviors and thoughts can be challenged not immediately, but on a graduated scale that can be dealt with effectively by the patient. Therefore, CBT and its main goals are easily met, unlike some therapies that require useless repetition without much positive gain.

COGNITIVE-BEHAVIORAL *ASSESSMENT MODEL

As with any therapy, assessment models exist to identify behaviors and or cognitive distortions. Almost all professionals in the mental health field have assessment models and/or assessment tools.

The tool used in CBT starts out with a typical assessment model, but with some unique steps that allow for identification immediately of some of the biggest and most prolific issues that are causing problems in the patient's life:

Step 1: Identify critical behaviors that are causing issues - here the model is simple and direct and asks questions as to what areas of life are most painful and/or causing dysfunction.

Step 2: Determine whether critical behaviors are excesses or deficits and what adjustments can be made - this is actually quite a large step and requires additional evaluation of what as an overview can elicit some initial ideas which can be investigated later (i.e. baseline).

Step 3: Evaluate critical behaviors for frequency, duration, or intensity (obtain a baseline as behavior modification suggests) as mentioned above, because of the importance of determining a baseline for a frequency of behaviors that are maladaptive and/or cognitive distortions which can be used later and paired together for possible therapy.

Step 4: If excess, attempt to decrease frequency, duration, or intensity of behaviors; if deficits, attempt to increase behaviors. Here you can clearly see possible ways to decrease the causation of maladaptive behaviors and/or cognitive distortions. This is typically where the therapist and the patient will work together to create an entire profile of events, a history including the impact that changes will have over time.

Step 5: Devise supporting reinforcement, extinction or suppression of disorders - here we see the influence of behavior modification by using supporting reinforcement and/or extinction or suppression of disorders. While this concept is not new, the inclusion of cognitive distortions along with behavior modification allows for the smoother flow of information and suggested therapy between patient and therapist. Behavioral models as well as new supporting Vogt and cognitions will be suggested to further reinforce the behavior modification model.

Even though this system, which is been cited as a source below, was created specifically for the purposes of an evaluation and or assessment tool, the author has added additional concepts. A blending of several schools is always best and is at the heart of CBT.

Further, we wish to reiterate the importance of a multi-dimensional approach when it comes to the combination of cognitive therapy, behavioral therapy and tying in important feelings and emotions during the entire process.

Feelings and emotions can fuel positive reinforcement as well as successive and graduated goals being achieved:

EFFECTIVE CONSIDERATIONS FOR THE ASSESSMENT

Once the assessment has been made, baselines have been taken, behavior modification suggested, as well as cognitive therapy introduced, we are now free to look at the larger picture because CBT involves many other aspects in a patient's life.

Treatment is best ***not done in a vacuum*** and should always involve people that are important to the patient. Even if the patient does not need to make all of the social criteria below part of his or her treatment, all of these aspects should be taken into consideration by the therapist and those that work on the treatment care plan:

- **Family & friends** - in order to preserve the integrity and privacy of the patient, the only family and friends involved should be the ones that are aware of the care plan. Here we also can involve people with just enough information to allow them to contribute their provided function. For example, a family member may only need to know that they wish to participate in a daily exercise to improve the person's mood and health, not that this item is actually ordered on a care plan.
- **Job/ workplace** - the only interaction that members at work should have with any patient should be in the form of stress reduction and should be done so carefully and cautiously through superiors. Changing job responsibilities slightly or moving the person to a new division that has less overall responsibility or a completely new way of doing work that would relieve prior anxieties of the patient could involve other peers. Despite most people's fears, this type of adjunct therapy is done frequently and quietly at most workplaces that offer the least restrictive environment for their workers.
- **Societal position** - the patient may have responsibilities in society such as sitting on a board, involvement with the local Chamber of Commerce, etc. Patients can temporarily step down or have another family member take up responsibilities or reduce the amount of time devoted to such societal positions.
- **Personality** - the strength of personality is also important because this dictates exactly how the patient will interact with other people. Personality distortions, once they are corrected, can alter the way the person perceives reality and the way other people perceive this new aspect of an older or emerging personality. This should always be done carefully and in steps

and should be discussed by the therapist and the patient for the best possible choices.
- **Personal beliefs** - religious and/or ethical beliefs almost always impact behavior and therefore, should be a source of strength and not something that is restrictive in nature unless the person is emerging from an oppressive cult-like religion that is at the center of their disorders. Again, this is a thought process for the therapist and the patient.
- **Professional beliefs** - some patients hold very strong professional beliefs that can impact their behavior. For example, OCD people are often compelled to behave in repetitive manners that once cured, may seem to reduce their overall effectiveness and could impact their job performance. Such professional beliefs should be carefully screened and checked prior to the institution of therapies that might disrupt job performance, or at the very least, they should be discussed and managed by the patient and therapist.
- **Other considerations** - there are numerous other considerations that can impact diagnostics and/or suggested therapies that should be part of an overall baseline and screening. The key is to establish a diagnostic snapshot that best allows the therapist to choose a course of action along with the patient who will also understand the importance is of managing the overall impact on their lives.

The key to understanding all of this is to realize that as therapy progresses people begin to change. The idea is to make the changes positive ones wherever possible and limit any type of negative impact on the person's overall life scheme.

Occasionally the importance of mental health far outweighs a person's current job, and after therapy, they may need to seek a different type or style of living contingent on the requirements for their new perspectives on health.

INTERVENTION & TREATMENT ANALYSIS

Both cognitive and behavioral therapy require an understanding as to the correct type of intervention and analysis for treatment based on events in someone's life.

In our last section, we mentioned several important aspects that must be considered so that proper assessment could be made prior to determining the best types of intervention and treatment.

Intervention and treatment analysis require that we understand the steps and considerations first and then determine the best approaches to this process.

Multiple treatments can and should be proposed based on:

- ✓ The best type of cognitive therapy.
- ✓ The best type of behavioral therapy.
- ✓ The best type of management of both the emotions and feelings during the other two therapies.

It is not the express goal of CBT to manage all aspects, all the time. Remember our main focus is on determining the best type of intervention first, after we take our baseline.

For example, Randy has constant panic attacks while he is in public and finds it difficult to talk to other people. The panic attacks happen anytime he is surrounded by people he does not know, and has to give an account of who he is or what he needs.

What most people would consider average everyday behavior, like going to the bank and withdrawing money, is an extremely awkward and difficult situation for Randy.

The therapist has proposed a form of systematic desensitization to teach him ways to learn how to deal with scenarios and situations of escalating stress.

This is a form of intervention and treatment analysis that the therapist has made. Such decisions should never be made in a vacuum, and require a firm baseline and understanding that this should be and is the best possible overall treatment.

Lacking sufficient background information, the beginning and/or intervention series requires several understandings:

- ✓ **What information has been accrued during the baseline** study that suggests the therapy or therapies that you wish to use are the best?
- ✓ **What type of psychosocial focus** should your therapy have, if any?
- ✓ **Should the therapy or therapies that you choose involve scenarios** that are painful yet necessary to help the potential patient through their disorders?
- ✓ **What social tools can you use** during an intervention and should the intervention be coupled with immediate therapy constructs? Why?
- ✓ **What will be the impact** of the therapy on the person's thinking, behavior, and feelings?
- ✓ **Is it necessary to invoke discomfort** during any of this process and how could this be avoided, if necessary? Should it be avoided at first?
- ✓ **What are some of the top pieces of literature** in the area and/or white papers suggesting based on your current situation as a therapist with the current patient that you have?
- ✓ **Do you require the use of other professionals** such as a drug addiction specialist, in order to reach a certain level of functioning to administer therapy?

All of these scenarios involve an understanding of exactly what you're going to do before you begin the use of any therapy, and if the intervention becomes confrontational or more passive in nature contingent on disorders.

The good news is that **simply changing cognition** can always be the first starting step before you begin to affect or impact behavior. Of course, this is contingent on a scenario in which behavior is not currently destructive and thus needs to be ceased immediately, such as hard-core alcoholism, drug abuse etc. Ultimately the term "intervention" need not be draconian in nature. Passive intervention can work just as well.

THE POWER OF CBT: REMOVAL OF ERRONEOUS THINKING

Therapists can now tap various behavioral models via the baseline information and use them to spot and reduce critical behaviors that are disturbing the client and causing breakdowns in thought reactive models.

In other words, now is the time for interventions based on assessment and to utilize top strategies with tools like thought stopping, passive confrontation and, cognitive modeling. In our next section, we will discuss in detail ways to deal with a variety of the top cognitive distortions that make people's lives significantly more difficult.

Understand that the main function of CBT is the removal of erroneous thinking. One of the best ways to attack this is to look for the most common cognitive distortions.

Erroneous thinking is the result of cognitive distortions plus possible misunderstandings based on feelings and emotions. The impact to the behavioral aspect is the end result of the cognitive distortions manifested into erroneous thinking that can also be linked with problematic feelings and emotions. Let us delve into this area of cognitive distortions and explain in detail the necessity for correcting erroneous thinking.

CHAPTER 4
COGNITIVE DISTORTIONS MADE WHOLE

One of the most understood functions of psychology is to **teach individuals the importance of changing their thinking and behavior**. What may seem normal behavior to someone suffering from a series of cognitive distortions can be quite bizarre and unusual to the average person.

For example let's discuss Mark, who has been taught since the beginning of his life that all people are inherently evil (including him) and the only way to avoid "hellfire and damnation" was to be a strict practitioner of his religious faith.

Such thoughts can be commonplace in unique scenarios that involve learned negativism, as well as the acceptance of related cognitive distortions which lead to what many of us would call erroneous thinking; even if Mark differs here.

For example, Mark believing that he is inherently evil, makes his life **very difficult** because he must constantly be on guard and overcritical of himself with everything that happens in his life or suffer condemnation and possible reprisals from church elders.

For example, Mark is driving a car down the road and the tire blows. The average person would simply perceive this to be as a possibility in life that could happen to anyone.

Yet Mark believes that he is evil and something that he did recently is now causing a possible punishment by God.

When something goes wrong in Mark's life, he perceives it to be an extension of some type of balancing scale based on (good) positive events or punishment (bad).

In Mark's case, as he goes to therapy he realizes that it is possible for negative events to happen to anyone and it is not likely anyone's fault.

One technique involving **thought stopping** teaches Mark that he can substitute negative or erroneous thoughts with positive ones, especially when there is no evidence that he's done anything wrong.

This is not meant to be any kind of moral judgment on religious values, but a way to help people suffering from emotional pain when clearly the cause is not their fault. Instead of believing everything he does is the result of being evil, he could rather look at events as simply an active opportunity to begin to heal his mind by more positive thinking.

"I got a flat tire because of something bad I did last week," could be changed to "I got a flat tire because there's construction nearby and somebody didn't clean up several sharp objects." This is a much more relevant and truthful response.

Cognitive distortions, therefore, are one of the leading focuses of proper cognitive therapy. Speaking with the client and providing tests including *isolating some of the biggest cognitive distortions,* should be the first steps that any therapist should consider.

Next, the focus should be on some of the most limiting cognitive distortions that cause the most pain and disruptions during a person's day.

For example, if a salesman who must speak with people all day long believes that someone is being difficult with him because they simply don't like him as a person, this is a **cognitive distortion** that could be patently false.

Of course, we must determine whether or not the cognitive distortion is, in fact, true or false or perhaps true sometimes.

Here is a list of some of the top cognitive distortions as discussed by several psychology papers and magazines. You should keep these in mind and we will focus on several of the absolute worst distortions that seem to have the highest impact on the most number of people:

Personalizing - someone does not like me personally so they're always being rude and obnoxious just to me. This can cause many problems in the workplace.

Underestimating ability - I'm not capable of doing that job or performing that function no matter what others think or say (i.e. I'm terrible at math).

Unyielding standards - I absolutely positively must behave in a certain way no matter what the situation dictates because I must always be correct or right.

Entitlement beliefs - I have a right to behave any way I choose because someone owes me something. (This particular cognitive distortion is becoming a huge problem in our society.)

Justification and moral licensing - I've worked very hard at something and therefore I have the right to behave any way I choose because I deserve it and "earned" it.

A world from your own viewpoint - here the cognitive distortion does not allow someone to see anything from someone else's viewpoint that violates a specific set of standards. For example, you believe people must be poor for a reason and it is always their fault.

Being overly self-critical as a motivational source – here we need to constantly criticize and force extremes regardless of the situation. For example, your friend won a gold medal in the Olympics for sprinting and still, you believe he needs your help to run faster.

Recognizing feelings are the cause of behavior but not the other way around - for example, I don't feel like exercising today because I'm tired, even though if you did exercise, eventually you would have more energy. Feelings govern all of your behavior instead of dealing with behavior and feelings as they arise.

'All or nothing' thinking – that 'either I will succeed or I will fail this month by gambling my rent money. If I don't always succeed I am an absolute failure.'

Always using feelings as a basis for judgment of self and others - for example, Melissa didn't smile at me today so she must be angry with me. I worked really hard yesterday with the boss and he didn't say thank you, so I must be terrible at my job.

Believing feelings will always be negative - no matter what I do I'm always going to feel bad and people will treat me poorly no matter what I do.

Cognitive labeling - this is where someone constantly judges others based on a singular event and then labels them. For example, my last boyfriend was a total loser because he wouldn't spend money on me.

Cognitive conformity - this is where you see everything exactly the same as everyone else around you, even when there is evidence to the contrary. Several of my coworkers don't like Steve so I must mistreat him as well even though he's never done anything wrong to me.

Blaming and or transferring feelings onto others - this is when someone sees something they do not like in another person that is actually something they do. They will then attack this behavior in another but not correct it in themselves. Bullies tend to be this way. So are people who cannot confront their own issues.

Failure to consider alternative explanations - here a person accepts the first and easiest thing to believe based on their emotions, feelings and core ethics regardless of the details. This has also been referred to as *cognitive dissonance* whereby someone can only accept things within the reality of their own beliefs.

Cognitive dissonance - a 'disconnect' that causes a person to only accept things that they are capable of understanding and not look beyond them or it will cause extreme discomfort and force them to challenge erroneous beliefs.

Assumed similarity and beliefs - here a person cannot see beyond the psychological limitations of their own ethics, thoughts, and beliefs and perceives everyone else as thinking the same way. For example, Joe does not believe in God so he perceives that no other logical person would believe in God either.

Over thinking and or analysis paralysis - here a person is constantly unable to solve problems because they must drastically over analyze every possible outcome.

Preferring only familiar things -a person wishes to surround him/herself completely with every aspect of life that they understand and do not wish to go outside of their comfort zone.

Excessive rigidity - a person believes they are incapable of making large changes in their lives and must adhere to a strict schedule for their own good or perceived good.

OVER-GENERALIZING, MAGNIFYING NEGATIVES, MINIMIZING POSITIVES AND CATASTROPHIZING

Self-defeating behavior and undermining are at the root of maladaptive behavior. The above cognitive distortions are among some of the worst and should each be discussed as their own category. Many people suffer from varying degrees of these cognitive distortions and should always be taken into consideration by any therapist:

Over-Generalizing – this cognitive distortion can result in significant errors when it comes to proper thinking and can cause a lot of issues in your client's life.

Overgeneralization typically causes you to draw faulty conclusions based on a singular example. The only benefit of over generalizations is to allow you to come to a quick decision, yet typically it will always be based on an erroneous conclusion.

For example, Mary is slightly overweight and hasn't been able to get a job even though she is skilled. She believes that people are not hiring her because she is fat. While there may be a small degree of truth to this, the overgeneralization could keep her from continuing to look for work and finding a high-paying job.

It is never a good idea to draw a singular conclusion based on one or two events that take place in your life.

For example, Joe was afraid of African-Americans because he had a negative encounter once, years ago. Even though Joe is surrounded by outgoing and friendly people that are also African-American, he tends to harbor feelings of resentment and fear that not only are preventing him from making new friends but are reducing the quality of life that he experiences.

It is important in life that you do not allow overgeneralization to completely control your behavior, but rather seek out new experiences and exceed your comfort zone in safe settings.

Magnifying negatives - this cognitive distortion tends to be in effect whenever we find ourselves surrounded by people that seem to be filled with gloom and doom. People also tend to always look on the negative side because this seems to make sense to their thinking.

For example, Lisa has had bad dating experiences with men and now believes that anytime she goes out on a date something bad will always happen.

For Lisa, even the smallest negative event becomes her fault and she believes that this is simply just the way things are. This causes a great deal of emotional distress for Lisa and now she tends to always see things as completely negative even if the smallest occurrence happens.

Of course, the people that are magnifying negatives also tend to minimize positive outcomes as well.

Minimizing positive outcomes - this is a common distortion where people will take good events and reduce them down to the bare-bones minimum so as to make them perceive themselves and others as less effective or incapable of having certain levels of success or enjoyment in life.

This form of *self-debasement* or *self-punishment* is common in people that have been highly criticized in their lives. There are times in our life we need to celebrate having success, but there are always those that believe no matter how positive an event is, something negative is just around the corner because of it.

Whether or not life has taught people to think this way certainly is worth discussion; however, in life, there are times when we must take the positive for exactly what it is.

Many people in varying degrees suffer this common type of cognitive distortion.

Catastrophizing - this cognitive distortion forces people into believing even the smallest negative event is something catastrophic in nature. Essentially this is when someone makes a mountain out of a molehill.

This type of individual finds it difficult to enjoy life to even the smallest degree because they're always awaiting the next dire event to take place in their life.

The above cognitive distortions are very much real and if you ask any therapist who's been practicing for any length of time, all of these are important and should be taken into consideration when attempting to create and eliminate many of these cognitive issues.

As part of your therapy, you will need to construct ways to effectively deal with some of the worst of these distortions by countering them with therapy.

This will not be easy especially for those that hold many negative views in life. Just getting someone to be somewhat optimistic could be a massive achievement on your part and it will require ongoing work as well as confrontational thinking in order to expose the cognitive distortions.

Take the opportunity to constantly confront negative thinking and try to have the patient or client visualize the exact opposite of what they're saying all the time.

Thought stopping is an effective tool, however it can only be so if the client perceives it as such.

Sometimes we have to admit defeat in certain areas of thought and shape different types of cognition that can actually work in a negative functional framework.

Utilizing negative functional frameworks with people that have severe cognitive distortions may be the first step towards moving towards more positive thought and redirecting them into a better place where they can achieve success in their lives and limit emotional disturbances.

REDUCING EMOTIONAL DISTRESS WITH CBT

Now that we've had a thorough discussion of some of the worst of the cognitive distortions that are causing emotional distress in people's lives, we need to discuss how to reduce that distress. You are already aware that we must first confront and deal effectively with cognitive distortions using thought stopping, mental frameworks and thought replacement as the first line of defense.

The next step for reducing emotional distress is to look into the client's own thinking and emotions and begin to show them that a person need not be controlled by negative thoughts and negative emotions.

One of the best ways to do this is through positive visualization exercises. Yes, positive visualization. Try it.

For example, Charlie (19) was beaten up a lot in high school and now he is afraid to hang out with other males his own age. Charlie always believes that when he gets around a group of other males, there's the potential that he will be beaten up again.

A clever therapist would eventually get Charlie into a group therapy session with other people his own age who have been through similar experiences.

At the very beginning, positive visualization can be used for Charlie as he can imagine himself in group therapy session with other boys his own age.

Again, systematic desensitization could be used to eventually get Charlie to confront his fears step by step.

The reduction in stress over time could be highly beneficial to Charlie and for other boys as well and even adults that have experienced similar situations.

The key point is to always counter the emotion with logic and common sense, giving examples of positive outcomes for other individuals that have had similar experiences.

The exciting part of CBT is that you can take into consideration not only the necessary tools to change cognitive distortions but you can also focus on the reduction in anxiety and other out-of-control emotions than can elicit negative behavior.

We can also take into consideration behavior modification tools and create situations where people like Charlie follow a self-motivational, self-reward set of steps.

Since Charlie is now 19, you must look towards his future potentially in college and at other events where he must gather with his peers. Therapy could be highly focused and not only change thoughts but modify emotions and eventually reward positive behavior in constructive group therapy sessions. Positive visualization becomes the doorway to all of this.

CHALLENGING MALADAPTIVE THOUGHTS & DESTROYING THEM

Our next step in dealing with the removal of cognitive distortions and restrictive emotions is to target maladaptive thoughts in a series of steps:

- ✓ First, identify the limiting and/or maladaptive thoughts that are linked to the corresponding cognitive distortions.
- ✓ Second, identify the pain and emotional turmoil that the cognitive distortions are causing.
- ✓ Third, target the appropriate counter therapy involving positive visualization, thought stopping, positive replacement of thoughts and possibly group therapy.

Identifying maladaptive thoughts is as easy as targeting cognitive distortions and working your way forward to see what behavior they cause. For example, we know that in Charlie's case, the fear of being physically beaten would keep him from becoming part of groups of his peers. Once the threat is reduced in his mind, he is much more likely to work towards being with a few people at a time and eventually with an entire group.

The key is to replace the maladaptive behavior with adaptive behavior. Yes, this will take time especially depending on how deep the maladaptive behavior is. Yet utilizing a variety of different tools can guarantee that over time, even people like Charlie can have a full recovery.

CHAPTER 5:
MODERN CBT & THE LATEST TOOLS

CBT can include a variety of combinations of helping tools (coping tools). This is because the therapy is focused on solutions, not endless sessions.

In addition, CBT offers unique aspects that give real life opportunities for patients to resolve current and future issues by themselves. Over the next few pages, were going to discuss some of the top tools via therapies that we can teach our clients as we guide them through the various tools necessary to heal any maladaptive behaviors and/or cognitive distortions.

These tools include:

- Systematic desensitization
- Exposure therapy
- Stress inoculation
- Cognitive processing
- Acceptance therapy
- Commitment therapy
- Mindful cognitive therapy
- Meditative practices
- Behavioral modification

Finally, there is real hope for people that are suffering, because once they have learned their own coping mechanisms, life will dramatically improve and allow them the opportunity to become healed and focused. Let's take a look at each of these tools now.

SYSTEMATIC DESENSITIZATION

We have given several examples of systematic desensitization in this guide as an exposure therapy. This is a 'confrontational' tool but it is used in a progressive manner in such a way so that at the conclusion of the timeframe given, the patient will be able to fully deal with something that truly has been causing them emotional distress.

For example, Steve is afraid of snakes and even the thought of a snake can cause a panic attack. Here, the therapist has devised a series of steps to allow Steve to eventually be able to *handle snakes* without having a panic attack:

1. Steve envisions what a snake looks like.
2. Steve is shown pictures of snakes.
3. Steve visits a zoo and looks at the snake exhibit.
4. Steve is invited to sit in the same room with snakes.
5. Steve looks at and eventually touches a single snake.
6. Steve handles several snakes for a brief time.
7. Steve spends part of the day working with an expert snake handler and handles snakes.
8. Steve is no longer afraid of snakes.

This is how ***systematic desensitization*** is typically structured over a certain time frame. The key components are that Steve is in the state of relaxation and reduced stress as he experiences each of these steps and is carefully monitored by his therapist. Steve can back out of any of the steps at any time, but in order to finally be deemed "cured" he must eventually complete all the steps.

EXPOSURE THERAPY

It should be stated that systematic desensitization is a form of exposure therapy. Exposure therapy is simply a way to help people confront their phobias based on the best possible outcome and what the therapist perceives as the most effective way for someone to overcome whatever is causing them emotional duress.

Exposure therapy can be used for a variety of situations including overcoming:

- ✓ Phobias of all kinds
- ✓ Obsessive-compulsive disorders
- ✓ Social anxiety disorders
- ✓ Post-traumatic stress disorders, and
- ✓ Anxiety orders of all kinds . . .

We list **social anxiety disorders** as its own separate category because this is a very common disorder and can easily be treated by using exposure therapy as a form of systematic desensitization.

There are a variety of different methodologies that are used with exposure therapy, and systematic desensitization is one of the most popular methods.

Of course, the ultimate goal is to get the patient to face their fears in a series of steps that help them overcome their phobia while reducing excessive anxiety.

Direct exposure is typically one of the fastest ways to recover from a phobia. However, it can cause panic attacks, extreme anxiety and other physiological reactions.

Contingent on what the client wants, what they are capable of tolerating and how quickly they wish to recover from a phobia, the therapist determines the type of exposure therapy that should be chosen. There is a wide range of different types of exposures that range from slight to extreme.

The reason for presenting systematic desensitization first was so that the reader could clearly see the benefits of a graduated or series of progressive steps that allow a person to handle the emotions and physiological reactions when being exposed to the phobia on a graduated scale.

It is always important that the therapist take the most careful control to ensure that you do not overwhelm your patient when choosing the right type of exposure stimuli.

Here **behavior modification** is useful because we can involve **extinction** through a series of systematic exposures to the point where the threat no longer is considered to be either relevant or even registers as a reactive stimulus. Ultimately exposure therapy has been scientifically proven to help people overcome phobias and should be strongly considered as a therapy that works as well as and with CBT.

STRESS INOCULATION

Stress Inoculation Therapy (SIT) is an effective psychotherapy that was designed to help patients deal with stressful situations by preparing in advance and being able to weather the storm of adverse stimuli and negative conditions throughout their day.

The therapy is based on **relapse prevention** techniques that allow someone to shore up their resistance to a specific set of stimuli. It is highly effective at helping people deal with stressful situations such as what you might experience at work or how to resist certain temptations such as alcohol, drugs etc. The therapy also educates and informs people about how to anticipate certain stressful situations and how to prepare for them in advance and de-escalate the stimuli's impact.

When a person has concluded stress inoculation, the patient knows that they can both anticipate and deal with a variety of stressful situations. This is highly effective therapy for people in stressful jobs such as police, fire, air traffic controllers or anyone who seeks to inoculate from stress and prepare to deal with stress in a realistic and intelligent way.

The therapy involves understanding when stressful situations will occur and the rehearsal of successfully dealing with the events related to negative stimuli.

COGNITIVE PROCESSING

Cognitive processing therapy (CPT) is best known as an effective therapy for dealing with events related to posttraumatic stress disorder.

It surmises that post-traumatic stress disorder (PTSD) is a very difficult disorder to recover from. PTSD generates **large amounts of negative emotions** and is difficult to cope with. PTSD can occur at almost any time and can be traumatic and difficult to cope with. Because of this, PTSD sufferers create **natural blocks** that make it difficult to overcome and eventually confront many of these negative emotions.

Cognitive processing incorporates trauma-specific cognitive techniques that allow patients to see actual sticking points and ways to overcome them using clear and logical thinking.

One effective way is to locate current triggers and work backward to the trauma. The therapist then asks the patient to recall events in this manner and the most vivid back to the least vivid, using coping points as tools.

The therapist then discusses how such triggers can be reduced once the aspect of the traumatic event is processed. Talking about how events happened and adding a conclusion to these events can be used to help remove blocks and allow the cognition a chance to be dealt with and then reduced in impact and finalized in the least traumatic method.

The main focus of the treatment takes the patient through differing ways to understand **how the traumatic event impacts their life** and things around them and ways to reduce the negative effects to their current life.

This is a highly intensive therapy but allows the patient to look back through events and organize them in a way that can be dealt with on not only an emotional level, but in an organized and thinking manner that delivers a reduction in stress and the ability to manage these thoughts.

The patient can then examine events by confronting them in a manner that is less emotional and allows them to draw conclusions that dissipate many of the symptoms and triggers. Automatic triggers are found and removed.

This therapy is highly productive for anyone that is been through traumatic experiences because it allows for long-term dissipation of negative emotions and for the person to eventually draw strength from the trauma that had taken place.

This also allows the patient to identify automatic thoughts and emotions that occur and eventually place them into different categories and reduce their impact on a person's life.

The process starts like this:

- ✓ The therapist discusses how PTSD / Trauma can be controlled and its impact reduced by learning how the trauma is causing dysfunction in the patient.
- ✓ The patient writes down how the trauma is causing life issues like guilt, depression and or other issues.
- ✓ The trauma is discussed and steps are taken to "process" it differently, using a kind of thought stopping and thought replacement where trauma causes mal adaptive issues until it is fixed.

Dire experiences such as military combat can then be regulated in a manner that can be controlled over time and allow the dissipation of difficult emotions.

The final phase allows the PTSD sufferer to begin to process the events of the trauma(s) in a systematic method that eventually will be used to restructure their lives in a positive manner.

Cognitive processing takes place during the entire therapy but the final steps allow for the PTSD sufferer to decide the best possible ways to deal with the negative events.

The therapist guides the patient on how to limit the impact of powerful *automatic occurring emotions* and events that replay in someone's mind until they are manageable.

The therapy can take about 12 weeks but is well worth the time, as treatment for trauma needs decompression and exploration as well as resolution. If someone has experienced a serious trauma, this is an excellent therapy and cognitive processing should be used especially over longer therapy sessions.

ACCEPTANCE THERAPY

Acceptance therapy or as it is sometimes referred to, **acceptance and commitment therapy** (ACT) is a relational therapy to CBT and is considered an intervention tool that focuses on mindfulness and the ability for a person to come to an acceptance ideology. For example, if a person is married and they've been cheating on their spouse and the other spouse is willing to have reconciliation, this therapy could be proposed as a possible intervention/ solution.

ACT has evolved over time and is now used to help people deal with difficult feelings and emotions and to have patients move towards valued behavior. The therapy teaches the importance of not overreacting, yet trying *not* to avoid unpleasant situations that are a necessity for growth.

ACT also envisions the use of truth as a methodology of mindfulness as well as the ability to focus on making choices *of one's own truth* that allow revelations and re-association with the acceptance of whom you truly are and how to make positive changes for the future.

The ACT teaches the importance of **gaining control of one's thoughts, feelings and emotions** and channeling all of this into something positive as a reflection of what a person should consider becoming. The therapy also stresses truth when it comes to finalizing all of these activities into a cohesive functional methodology and ideology that allows for growth and control in one's life.

MINDFULNESS-BASED COGNITIVE THERAPY

Mindfulness-based cognitive therapy (MBCT), similar to acceptance therapy, is an approach created as a form of relapse prevention. Research indicates that it is particularly effective for people dealing with the major depressive disorder (MDD) and other related depressive issues.

There are similar therapies such as mindfulness-based stress reduction (MBSR) that are also effective, but mindfulness-based cognitive therapy (MBCT) is an extension of cognitive behavioral therapy (CBT).

The therapy stresses Eastern psychological strategies that include meditation. The patient is also educated about the causations of depression and how proper meditation can bring someone to a point to where depression and its impacts can be greatly reduced and/ or controlled.

Part of the philosophy directs individuals to also learn acceptance and mindfulness so as to focus on all incoming thoughts and learn about the feelings that are caused.

With mindfulness, you are completely aware of ways to begin to control the thoughts that cause negative emotions. The process has been referred to as "de-centering" by disengaging oneself from overly critical thoughts and emotions. Essentially you are striving for complete calm, much the way a Buddhist might attain knowledge of the self through proper meditation.

Eastern philosophies have always promoted strong and beneficial meditative practices that teach the removal of one's self from the center of the whirlwind of emotions.

The key is not to react to negative thinking patterns but rather become more philosophical about the life of the events within life and ***that all beings are in need of understanding*** of life and how it functions.

MBCT therefore understands functions via the etiological theory that when depression occurs, automatic cognitive processes can be triggered which thereby causes depressive episodes. Meditative processes can counter this.

By disrupting this pattern, removing the self and remaining focused on and mindful of these thoughts, the automatic triggering of depressive episodes can be neutralized.

The key is to have these thoughts without judgment and determine their origin and then rethink notions as to why such thoughts and thought patterns are occurring.

Therefore, the goal was **to interrupt automatic triggers that cause depression** and help the individual to no longer have depressive episodes.

Observed clinical outcomes have proven time and time again that MBCT as an extension of mindfulness allows for drastic improvement in depressive episodes and can eliminate depression over time.

MEDITATIVE PRACTICES

So now you've seen the benefit of several different types of mindfulness therapies. Many are linked to meditative practices, especially when the function is to reveal and/or isolate and eventually remove automatic triggers that cause:

- ✓ Depressive episodes
- ✓ Anxiety attacks
- ✓ Mood swings
- ✓ Overeating, or
- ✓ Relapses to drugs or alcohol.

Meditative practices when guided by professionals can also help you to establish a core understanding of not only the self but the higher self as well.

While some Western philosophies discourage Eastern practices, mounting evidence is showing the importance of daily meditation and the positives are adding up quickly.

Not only can you refocus vital energies, but you can also **continue to grow emotionally** and learn to control as well as modify the way you react physiologically and emotionally to events in your life. Biofeedback techniques also are an extension of meditative philosophies and have been shown to offer many different types of physical as well as mental benefits, so please consider looking into meditative practices for you and your patient.

BEHAVIORAL MODIFICATION (R+)

Behavior modification has been discussed in several locations in this guide and we also wish to point out that there are many different tools that can be used to help other types of therapy become successful.

Wherever there is repetition (i.e. eating, drinking, consumption of drugs, OCD etc.), there is an opportunity for behavior modification to have an impact.

Practitioners of behavior modification understand its power and the ability to reinforce an alternative behavior or remove behavior by shaping and eventually molding this behavior to cease to exist. Both are goals that will help patients.

For example, during the course of a PTSD treatment, the therapist suggests that every time Stephen can control the shakes and tremors, that he rewards himself with a small treat such as a piece of chocolate, which he loves.

While this may seem silly, behaviorists understand the power of positive reinforcement so that eventually good behavior will be repeated simply because *it is good behavior* and not just because it is reinforced.

Intermittent reinforcement eventually can become ***ongoing reinforcement through other types of reward-based systems.*** For example, going from chocolate *every* time that the tremors stop, to every third time and eventually to just a feeling of positive wellbeing should be the final goal.

Behavior modification also has the ability to reinforce almost any other kind of therapy.

Behaviorists believe that behavior modification alone can change behavior; however, CBT is the inclusion of behavioral techniques along with shaping and molding of thoughts and emotions. The two are not mutually exclusive.

Obviously, **when all three come together**, they are at their best, and this is why combined therapy sessions can typically achieve considerable results much faster than only one of the therapies.

By combining cognitive practices with behavior modification and mindfulness, you have a very effective therapy that can remove the patient from the maelstrom of competing thoughts and negative energy and place them at a point where they begin to control the outcome of their life.

The key is to take CBT to the maximum level by invoking effective cognitive therapy, mindfulness, controlling thoughts with emotions, and the behaviorist model of a reward- based economy directed to oneself.

This is also the key to understanding and expression of CBT because ultimately a therapist should be more concerned about the tools necessary to completely allow the patient to gain control over their lives, without the necessity for the patient to constantly return to the therapist's chair.

We will discuss in our next section the six phases of CBT and how all of this comes together.

CHAPTER 6:
THE 6 PHASES OF CBT EXPLAINED FOR THERAPY USE

Up to and including this point, we have seen CBT broken down into its component parts and various explorations of different psychological tools and the implementation of each of these tools as additional potential therapies.

The active use of CBT has been broken down into six different phases, some of which we have briefly touched upon and yet others we wish to expand upon in new and exciting ways that will benefit not only therapists, but the patients that will be on the receiving end.

Here are the phases that we will be discussing in each individualized section:

1. Assessment or psychological assessment revisited
2. Re-conceptualization as further cognition
3. Skills acquisition for the patient
4. Skills consolidation and application training
5. Generalization and maintenance for the patient
6. Post-treatment assessment follow-up

ASSESSMENT OR PSYCHOLOGICAL ASSESSMENT

Earlier in the guide we discussed the DSM (V) and the importance of using it as a tool for psychological assessment.

Obviously, this is the main tool that we use to determine what disorders are troubling to the patient, but one thing that we did not discuss was one of the best ways to use this information **to** *further predict the needs of the client*.

For example, if the DSM suggests that a person is suffering from social anxiety disorder, what the DSM does not suggest are the correct and necessary countering therapies that could be chosen (typically).

Before we can actually choose the therapy, we must understand the implications of:

- ✓ **Additional underlying diagnoses** that may need to be taken into consideration for maximum effect,
- ✓ **How additional underlying diagnoses** will affect the correct treatment regimen and why, and
- ✓ **The best possible steps for making the patient aware of** and involving them in the treatment.

Remember that CBT requires that we *involve the patient* and provide them with an active set of steps, values and interactive information as well as additional homework to help them recover in an effective manner. For example, social anxiety disorder will require the patient to provide detailed information about when certain triggers cause the anxiety attacks and/or possible panic attacks.

As we know, behavior modification is a powerful part of recognizing exactly when and how these triggers can take place. When we combine cognitive therapy with identifying triggers, then we have the necessary information to focus on the correct treatment steps.

In addition, psychological assessment requires that you *look beyond just triggers and triggering events* to the actual causation of why the triggers were implanted in the first place. This could require subconscious precursors to be revealed, even if you only focus on conscious constructs.

This is a critical piece of information that typically is not revealed initially during any type of assessment, but must be kept first and foremost within the understanding of the therapist and as to the correct time for its revelation.

Of course, **the revelation is contingent upon what is best for the patient**; however, if a simple trigger can be identified, it should immediately be provided to the patient. Considerations of any assessment must always consider what is best for the patient and the resolution of whatever disorder they are suffering from, **especially the cessation of anxiety-producing situations such as a panic attack**. Later cognitive therapy can also be used to remove the triggering event.

RE-CONCEPTUALIZATION

Many therapists who practice CBT consider this phase to be where the patient is able to re-conceptualize events that are taking place in their life in a way that creates the triad: thoughts, feelings and emotions and their resultant behavior.

One aspect of CBT is to take the patient by the hand and let them experience each of the three elements of the triad, but from different perspectives like the therapist does.

For example, the patient might experience a very powerful feeling that also makes them very sad, such as the death of a loved one or close friend.

Re-conceptualization might redirect them to thinking about such an event in a positive way. This is especially true if you can combine certain ethics or philosophies that the patient holds in high regard, such as a religious belief.

For example, Omar believes in reincarnation and that people that are good reincarnate to higher levels of consciousness and live better lives when they are reborn.

Omar is sad at the passing of his brother, but the therapist reminds him that instead of being sad that he should also consider the passing of a loved one, especially someone like his brother who lived a good life, as also a celebration based on his religious ethics and values.

This is at the core of re-conceptualization. The same process can be used regardless of the person's ethics, religion or values. Use this to help patients see sad events from another angle.

Taking an individual by the hand and looking at their thoughts, which can also be expressed in ways that they may never have considered, can aid in the therapy as well.

For example, Joe thinks that he is incapable of losing weight because every time that he tries, he fails. After intensive psychotherapy, it is learned that Joe has been dealing with anger issues and is quite literally swallowing his aggression in the form of food.

Once Joe was freed of the aggressive and bothersome thoughts, he now has been given a new lease on life because he no longer is turning his aggression inward and harming himself. The triggering event was resolved.

The same can be said for dealing with abnormal behavior. We've seen the benefits of behavior modification especially if they can be linked to thoughts and feelings.

The triad allows us to explore and re-conceptualize ways for patients to find their way out of the maze of their own thoughts, feelings, and emotions.

A good therapist will always find ways to redirect their patients by utilizing relevant personal ethics, values, beliefs, feelings and behaviors. Always keep the therapy centered on these things and you will have success with any patient that you are attempting to help this way.

SKILLS ACQUISITION

Skills acquisition assumes that based on the current scenario of your patient, that they are lacking somewhere. The patient is dealing with relevant thoughts, feelings, and emotions and/or negative behavior without coping tools.

It is your job to take a baseline of exactly what is going on, much like a snapshot in time that can be used as a roadmap to determine what skills are necessary but lacking in the patient.

Skills acquisition need not be anything burdensome or labor-intensive. It could be something as simple as a behavior chart based on intermittent reinforcement combined with thought stopping and thought replacement.

Perhaps the skills necessary for the patient to continue to grow might be meditation and mindfulness directives combined with positive reinforcement when they choose good behavior over bad. Create the model they need.

Interestingly enough there may be situations where patients need to unlearn mal-adaptive skills through extinction.

Remember that we always reinforce the behavior that we wish to do over and over. If that behavior is also self-reinforcing, like eating Oreo cookies and the pleasure it invokes, then we must determine the removal of primary reinforcers that are keeping negative behavior alive. This is also an important part of skills acquisition. Often, we must unlearn the things that we have learned as a skill too.

SKILLS CONSOLIDATION AND APPLICATION TRAINING

No skills are learned in a vacuum. Once we see the deficits, we must then **compile the correct skills and consolidate them** to give us the best overall view of the patient and how they will be able to cope and eventually become high functioning again.

We then need to take time to train the patient on the appropriate steps to take, especially if these are new skills or hampering skills that we must remove in order to have a positive impact.

Consolidating skills also allows us to focus on the least number of tools necessary to complete the job.

For example, if simply allowing the patient to meditate could alleviate many of the negative triggers that are occurring in their life, this would be a good first place to start as long as application training is also being considered.

No patient should attempt any type of skills without directives and ongoing monitoring from the therapist.

As we teach patients ways to cope and better coping mechanisms, we must be there if things break down or there are relapses. We need to explain to our patients that sometimes this is just part of the process and that learning and mastering a new skill can take time.

Application training demands that we be highly vigilant as therapists and make sure that the patient is utilizing coping mechanisms and/or skills in a manner that is conducive to their abilities and their understanding of the impact upon their mental health.

Further, application training insists that there be goals set and that it is wise to keep a written journal of daily events to present at the next therapy session.

Application training also must be *mirrored by professionals* in a manner that is most easily understood, but with the same capability or nearly the same capability that the therapist demonstrates.

For example, the replacement of negative thoughts with positive ones must be fully explained in a manner that makes sense to the patient and not just the therapist.

Involving yourself in ongoing **therapy training** of the patient is not only a requirement for being a good therapist, but is absolutely essential for skills assessment and consolidation. You may be required to take phone calls at unusual times, especially if the patient has any dissociative issues or needs additional coaching through difficult new events.

Ultimately it is your goal to provide the best possible set of tools that are least intrusive in someone's life, while still providing the necessary information for them to consolidate and then utilize these tools in an effective manner to continue their mental health growth.

GENERALIZATION AND MAINTENANCE

Generalization and maintenance happen when skills and tools and coping mechanisms come together in a manner that allows a complete understanding of functionality and form.

In this phase, the patient has become used to the tools necessary to effect change and improve their current mental health.

It is at this point that the therapist can gloss over some of these tools and techniques and focus solely on maintenance.

For example, in behavior modification, once a primary reinforcer has been effective in shaping behavior, it can be shifted to intermittent reinforcement. This is a form of maintenance that allows the behavior to continue with the least amount of effort necessary.

Generalization and maintenance as an exploration by both the therapist and the patient have come to the conclusion that the tools that they are using are effective.

When this happens, maintenance becomes the main goal, but one must also keep a close eye on the changes in thoughts, emotions, and behavior.

Should relapse or other events occur, it will require another session with the therapist to reestablish this phase. This is a delicate step to post-treatment and follow-up.

POST-TREATMENT ASSESSMENT FOLLOW-UP

Once we have passed generalization and entered into the maintenance phase, it is time for the patient to enter post treatment.

Keep in mind that the patient is not yet completely free of the disorder, but rather will require additional follow-up to make sure that the treatment has been effective.

This is why the prior step of generalization and maintenance is necessary to determine whether or not the patient can enter post-treatment.

Consider this a checkup several months down the road to make sure that the treatment was effective and that the tools that are being used by the patient are still operating with efficiency. You can also evaluate the tools' performance.

The therapist may be required to make additional tweaks and adjustments where small alterations as a form of post-treatment are necessary but do not require another session.

Having an assessment and/or follow-up will determine based on the DSM whether or not there is a potential for relapse or if the patient appears to be under control or "cured." Make sure you refer to all of your notes and carefully assess the patient as they may wish not to resume treatment in the case of a relapse.

Also, keep in mind during your assessment that you look for any telltale signs that the patient is attempting to conceal or hide any and/or all of the disorders that have been initially revealed.

Where there is resistance by the patient, that's the best time for you to consider re-examining the situation and if it is revealed to you that the patient is still suffering, you should suggest returning to treatment and sessions.

Additional assessment tools may be necessary to pinpoint where weaknesses occurred during the treatment or whether or not the patient simply lost control.

It is also possible that once you've established a new baseline, that you are simply dealing with matters that are briefly resurging but will eventually subside.

Look for old triggers and events that could have been the cause of these issues as sometimes therapy may relocate or redirect the possible cause of a relapse.

It is possible also that a therapist may have missed other telltale signs during the course of therapy that they've been involved with, so here is a time to finalize and completely remove any final obstacles to the patient's mental health.

Remember that multiple sessions may be possible and you may have to work in differing venues to achieve maximum results, especially with multiple therapies like CBT. Never be afraid to ask the patient to return to therapy explaining that they are almost there but need a few more sessions.

CHAPTER 7:
BEST USES FOR CBT & BEYOND

Now you should be fully aware of the broad ranges of treatment that CBT can be used for and how you can quickly establish a variety of treatment options for many of the symptoms listed below:

- ✓ **Anger issues and anger management** - CBT is effective because it holds not only thoughts, but behavior and emotions to account. Anger issues can be quickly quelled by teaching mindfulness combined with behavior modification and the suppression of negative thought.
- ✓ **Anxiety problems** - there are many different types of anxiety disorders that can be quickly controlled because CBT works on the root causes and triggers of anxiety efficiently.
- ✓ **Panic attacks** - panic attacks can actually make a person feel like they might be dying and are very intense. Understanding the root causes of triggers and ways to suppress and eventually eliminate them is of great value to anyone suffering.
- ✓ **Dysfunctional issues** - the list is extensive here and CBT can help all kinds of dysfunctional issues especially as they relate to children, teenagers, and adults.
- ✓ **Childhood problems** - many people suffer from childhood problems well into adulthood especially when they deal with abusive homes, anxiety related issues and improper nurturing that can occur at the hands of abusive or poor parents. CBT can tackle the core causes and allow a person to deal with this trauma in a powerful and effective way.
- ✓ **Depression** - mindfulness training as well as the ability to refocus one's thoughts, feelings and emotions is a powerful tool that CBT offers to people who are suffering from depressive

issues. Few therapies have such a high degree of success and depression need not be a lasting disorder.
- ✓ **Addictive issues like drugs & alcohol** - the true strength of CBT is expressed in its ability to relieve people of the need for addictive drugs and/or alcohol or even addictive behaviors. Because we combine the complete spectrum of emotions, behavior and thinking, we are able to affect events in a person's life and also to prevent relapses.
- ✓ **Eating disorders** - behavior modification along with identification of eating triggers is a powerful tool that CBT can present in any situation. This even includes the addictive personality and how to deal effectively with it and to deprogram these triggers.
- ✓ **Health issues that cause psychological disorders** - many people suffer from a variety of health disorders that also can relate to mental health issues, such as obesity. The powerful combination of behavior modification along with the ability to reprogram how we think and then allow us to grow our emotions in a positive manner can help solve many common health issues and allow us to regain control.
- ✓ **Mood swings** – can be a form of the depressive disorder, however, mood swings are much more common and are equivalent to issues relating to bipolar disorder. Here, imbalances can be corrected using behavior modification (i.e. diet, meds.) and the focus can be directed to mindful therapy and meditative practices to help control volatile emotions.
- ✓ **Obsessive-compulsive disorder (OCD)** - interestingly enough OCD can be controlled through behavior modification and more mindful focuses. Helping someone to reduce the instances of repetitive negative behavior and to focus on growth towards other productive uses of their time is a primary function of CBT.
- ✓ **Phobias of all kinds** - exposure therapy along with behavior modification and cognitive therapy come together to quickly eliminate phobias of all kinds. CBT works wonders here because

all elements are brought to bear and fears can be made extinct quickly.
- ✓ **Post-traumatic stress disorder** - we have also explained in detail how CBT is highly effective at allowing people suffering from PTSD to eventually recover completely and view the events of their trauma in a new light.
- ✓ **Sexual and relationship problems** - acceptance therapy as an extension of CBT along with mindfulness can teach people with relationship and sexual disorder problems how to not only cope, but relearn the importance of connecting with their mate.
- ✓ **Sleep problems** - as an extension CBT would teach the importance of regular exercise as well as necessary sleep patterns to maintain good health. The importance of regular sleep is inculcated into the person going through the therapy.

Please keep in mind this is only a partial list of some of the top mental health disorders that plague our society that CBT is effective at dealing with.

As a therapist or even a layperson, it is up to you to make the proper decisions necessary to determine what aspect of CBT works best for what situation.

As always, competent therapists are necessary especially those trained in CBT to continue moving forward and to use the therapy because it is highly effective, and can be used in the least amount of time necessary to effect the greatest change.

Take the opportunity to consider the best extension of CBT therapy for you, your practice and of course your patients.

CONCLUSION

In this amazing guide, we have explored **Cognitive Behavioral Therapy** in a whole new light while emphasizing some of the key components necessary to practice it successfully.

Therapists should take a look at some of the new possibilities and the additional capabilities that CBT can bring to bear in any practice or setting.

If even one of the ideas in this guide sparks your imagination and allows you to structure new and more practical types of therapy, consider adding this to the pool of white papers that are constantly supporting and revitalizing CBT as perhaps one of the only essential therapies in dealing with the most generalized mental health issues.

Our goal here today has been to take a new look at combining therapies into a more generalized one-size-fits-all as long as that one size comes with additional benefits.

CBT is perhaps one of the best overall therapies because it **packs in all three levels necessary to effect positive change in almost any patient.**

We know the importance of involving a patient's thoughts, behaviors and emotions together to paint a complete picture of exactly what is necessary to help that patient through the difficult times in their life.

What people need today is not overly critical or endless lectures about ways to change their behavior, but practical tools that anyone can be taught to use easily so that they can not only correct disorders themselves, but eventually help themselves again in the future.

The good news about CBT is that it can also be taught to other people, even average and uneducated folks, as long as they understand the basics of altering negative for the positive.

While it also very critical to always have competent professionals to guide you through the practices of CBT, a patient that has had the opportunity to understand and learn effective tools can not only maintain their own mental health, but can teach these tools to their friends and family.

Please strongly consider using CBT not only in your practice but also in your daily life. As an expression of your belief in CBT, the utilization of the tools to maintain your own mental health should be practiced and practiced well.

Best Regards,
Bill Andrews

More books by Bill Andrews on this series can be found here-
https://geni.us/billbooks

FREE TRAINING

Thank you for reading this book. As a way of showing my appreciation, I want to give you a **5 Day Training program absolutely FREE** along with this book.

Free Training Reveals Step-By-Step...

How To Eliminate Stress, Anxiety & Depression Naturally From Your Life Forever...

Go To Below URL For Instant Access

https://bit.ly/cbt_depressiontraining

Printed in Great Britain
by Amazon